1200 Calorie Diet

How to quickly burn stubborn fat while enjoying delicious food without suffering through hunger | Easy and flavorful recipes that are high in protein and low in fat

Table of Contents

Introduction

Hey! Are you here because this title grabbed your attention? Search no more! Your hands are finally on the right book. Explore these extremely fun and nutritious recipes that promise to help you lose weight while keeping the fun and taste intact.

This book revolves around the widely relied on and promised diet plan with a high protein and low-fat content. Enjoy this meal plan, which has been recommended by many health professionals and depends on people looking forward to maintaining a healthy weight. You will receive the most delicious meal plan with the fewest calories, the least fat, and the highest protein content.

This looks to be one of the most dependable plans for suppressing cravings while also making you feel full and satisfied. Believe it or not, this will work wonders in helping you in your weight loss journey without depriving you of yummy food. Burning that stubborn fat is not going to be an issue anymore.

What are you waiting for then? This is it! This is the meal plan that your body needs.

Chapter 1: Calorie Deficit and Weight Loss

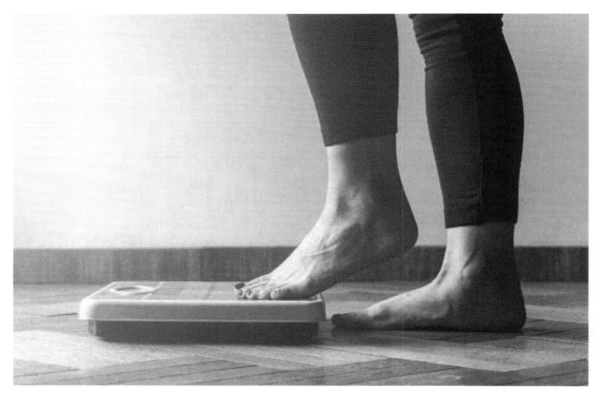

Start where you are. Use what you have. Do what you can!

In terms of weight loss, you must eat fewer calories per day or week than your body needs to keep your current weight. A gradual reduction in calories can result in weight loss.

As our lifestyles grow more and more physically sedentary, weight gain is becoming more common in the population. Eating without thinking, not exercising, being anxious, dealing with worldly demands, and sitting for long periods contribute to weight gain.

Before digging into the relationship between calorie deficit and weight reduction, it is critical to understand what calorie deficit is in the first place. To follow this diet, you must understand the concept of a calorie deficit and how it relates to weight loss and remain genuine and committed to your weight loss goals throughout your journey. The state of having consumed fewer calories than you have burned is referred to as being in an "energy deficit." One of the reasons it is referred to as an energy deficit is that calories are regarded as a unit of heat and energy. However, the term "calorie deficit" has been the center of attention for quite some time now because it is critical in losing and maintaining weight.

Remember! This may not be as straightforward as it appears. You shouldn't have to go hungry or spend several hours exercising to lose weight; in fact, there are several clever strategies you can use to lose weight while still satisfying your taste preferences. Let's talk about some of the modifications you may make to achieve a calorie deficit.

If you want to reduce your portion size, you'll also need to cut back on snacking. Consuming low-calorie foods at mealtime can aid in weight loss. As a natural outcome, you'll ingest fewer calories per day, eventually reaching the bottom of the calorie deficit diet spectrum.

Another method of achieving the calorie deficit goal is through physical activity. Suppose you improve your physical activity level, and by that, I mean your exercise and non-exercise movements. In that case, your risk of heart disease will be reduced. When you increase your activity level while maintaining your calorie intake, your body enters a calorie deficit, which means you will lose weight. Although you will burn more calories, your calorie intake will remain constant. While it may appear simple, remember that perseverance is the key to achieving any goal. It will only become instinctive if you do it on a consistent basis.

A recent study concluded that a combination of a low-calorie diet and regular exercise would significantly aid in weight loss and, more importantly, will aid in sustaining the weight loss achieved. The key to maintaining your weight is to consistently adhere to your diet and engage in regular physical activity, resulting in a calorie deficit in both directions.

Moreover, it is possible to estimate how many calories an individual burns daily in several ways.

For instance, you can use a physical calorie counter or an internet one to figure out how many calories they need each day. Moderately active people can estimate their daily calorie needs by multiplying their current body weight by 15.

Subtract 500 calories from that figure to get a rough estimate of how many calories one should consume for a healthy calorie deficit. Eating too few calories can also be unsafe. In addition, regular physical activity can help to create a calorie deficit.

Chapter 2: Dense, Low-Calorie Food

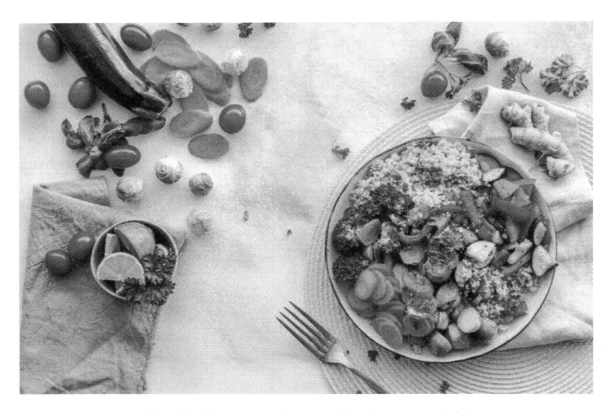

You don't have to eat less; you just have to eat right!

Understanding how calorie density affects one's diet, weight, and physical state is critical for making weight-loss changes.

The best thing about low-calorie dense food is that you don't have to restrict your intake and go hungry. Instead, make absolutely sure that every dish you eat is low in calories. This way, you can eat a large meal while still losing weight. Isn't this just a fantasy come true?

There's another way to understand this theory. A vegetable with 40 calories per 100 grams has a low-calorie density, whereas a chocolate muffin with 600 calories per 100 grams has a relatively very high-calorie count or calorie density.

Here, we will mention some healthy foods that have high nutritional value and are low on the caloric spectrum.

Vegetables

Green leafy vegetables are low in calories because they are mostly water and have a low carbohydrate and fiber content.

Lean Meat and Fish

Proteins like chicken, fish, turkey, etc., fall under the low-calorie density category. However, fattier meals and some fish have high-calorie density, so it is important to check and educate yourself on the caloric nature of the food.

Milk and Yogurt

This is an excellent source of protein. There is now a wide variety of fat-free and low-calorie milk available. A protein alternative is to use sugar-free yogurt. It contains a lot of protein. One cup (245 g) of plain yogurt made with whole milk contains approximately 8.45 g of protein.

Starchy Carbs

Starchy carbs may look like they are dense in calories, but once they are brought to heat and cooked, they fill up with water and reduce calories. Potatoes and other root vegetables are best in this regard.

Fruits

Fruits are high in fiber and water. Fruits have a low-calorie density, so try to incorporate them into the majority of your diet. You must eat lesser calories to lose weight, but not necessarily eat less. Fruits have high fiber content and a low-calorie count, so they can be used to replace high-calorie foods in our diet, allowing us to feel full and satisfied while consuming fewer calories. With fruit in breakfast cereals, we can reduce portion size and thus calories without feeling deprived. Fruits can also help us lose weight by replacing foods with a high glycemic index in our diet. So, it is recommended that you consume five servings of fruits per day, in various colors.

Sugar-Free Drinks

Sugar-free drinks work best at keeping you full and energetic. Be it water, your favorite coffee, or tea, all of these are low in calorie density and help you with hunger and weight loss.

Chapter 3: Food with High Volume

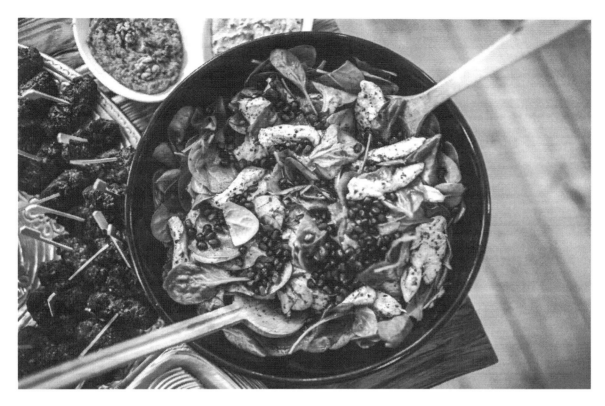

It's like hitting the jackpot when it comes to losing weight by consuming more food. There are several methods for increasing the number of nutrients in your diet, but one of the most effective is to eat more food in general.

Substituting higher-volume, lower-caloric foods for some of your high-calorie meal options will assist you in maintaining your calorie deficit while preventing hunger.

Rather than fixating on how many calories you consume, consider the quality of the food you consume. Having perfected this skill, consuming big quantities of food becomes second nature.

Instead of high-calorie foods, eat a wider variety of low-calorie, nutrient-dense foods. Volume eating is a technique rather than a diet or set of rules to follow. Simple strategies, such as carefully incorporating large amounts of low-calorie items into your diet, will help with weight loss more quickly and easily than you might think. As a result, you will be able to consume fewer calories while remaining satisfied.

Processed foods, such as cereal bars, chips, and soft drinks, account for the vast bulk of the high-calorie items available in the typical diet. These may look delicious, but they contain a significant quantity of calories for such a tiny amount of food. Aside from that, their nutritional benefits appear to be significantly smaller in most cases.

Vegetables

Loading up on vegetables is the quickest and easiest way to consume more food while burning fewer calories. Leafy greens have a higher fiber and water content per calorie than other foods. Including several cups of leafy greens in your diet daily will not affect your calorie intake.

A cup of granola, for example, has fewer than 20 calories but adds a significant amount of bulk to your plate, making you feel satisfied. In addition to these high-volume, low-calorie leafy greens, there are other options such as kale, which has 8.1 calories per cup. In contrast, spinach has 2.4 calories, or iceberg lettuce, around 8 calories per cup, whereas cabbage has 22 calories.

Whole Wheat

According to Jaramillo (a healthcare expert), switching from refined grains to whole grains will allow you to boost the volume of your meal by a significant amount. Whole grains provide a variety of minerals, including fiber, iron, and magnesium, among others. Whole grains also contain more fiber than processed grains.

Whole grain oats, brown rice, barley, and millet are all good choices for whole-grain diets since they have no more than 150 calories per half-cup of the grain they contain. Isn't that incredible?

Protein

Beyond the fact that leaner proteins are lower in fat and calories, they also allow for larger consumption of protein in comparison to their fattier counterparts. Reduce your intake of red meat and whole milk products while increasing your intake of chicken breasts, fish such as tuna and salmon, low-fat and unsweetened yogurt, cottage cheese, ground turkey, and other foods with less than 150-200 calories per cup.

Now, let's look at some of the incredible benefits of eating large amounts of high-volume meals. To begin, eating large amounts of high-volume meals has been shown to aid weight loss.

Replacing large amounts of lower-calorie food for small amounts of higher-calorie food results in increased food intake at a lower calorie cost, which in most cases benefits weight loss. When you are on a calorie-restricted diet, you will experience more pleasure. Hunger pangs will occur occasionally, but the more food you eat, the easier it will be to stick to your diet plan.

Fiber is a vital component that can only be gained via eating fuller meals. As shown by a research paper published in October 2019 in The Journal of Nutrition, fiber not only helps you feel full after eating, but it may also help you lose weight and maintain diet compliance. A study of the effects of various diets on 345 people discovered that fiber intake correctly predicted weight loss in those who participated in the trial.

Increasing the number of meals you eat will also provide more nutrition. In general, high-volume meals like leafy greens and lean proteins have more vitamins and minerals than low-volume foods like processed foods, typically higher in calories.

Chapter 4: Water

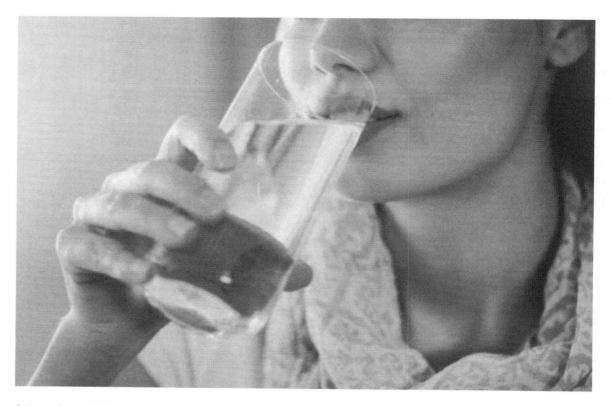

No one claims that drinking water before bed will make you lose weight, but research shows it does. Because water makes up 60% of your body, it plays a part in almost every biological function. Once your body is hydrated, it can perform tasks like thinking and fat-burning more effectively.

Water may aid in weight loss in a variety of ways. It may help you lose weight by suppressing your appetite, increasing your metabolism, and making exercise more efficient. While many variables, actions, and predispositions influence your body weight, staying hydrated may be a good place to start for long-term, modest weight loss.

Your initial instinct may be to find food when you're hungry. Food isn't always the answer. "The brain often confuses thirst, which is caused by moderate dehydration, with hunger," explains Melina Jampolis, MD, a board-certified medical nutritionist. "Drinking water may help reduce appetite if you are deficient in water, not calories." It promotes satiation by swiftly passing through the system and extending the stomach. It tells your brain you're full.

"Consuming water just before eating may assist lower food intake," says Elizabeth Huggins, a Registered Dietitian Nutritionist at Hilton Head Health. A 2016 study found that those who drank two glasses of water before a meal ate 22% less than those who didn't.

Another intriguing finding was that after an eight-week study, 50 overweight females who drank two glasses of water thirty minutes before meals without making any other dietary changes lost weight and had lower BMI and body composition scores.

Because water has no calories, drinking it instead of juice, soda, sweetened tea, or coffee can lower your overall liquid calorie consumption.   Choosing water over a 20-ounce soft drink saves you 250 calories.

Another pre-existing data in The American Journal of Nutrition claimed that overweight and obese women who drank water instead of diet drinks lost more weight throughout the weight-loss program. Water drinkers lost more weight than non-drinkers.

However, researchers argue that water is essential to all cellular activities in our bodies, from head to toe. Keep yourself hydrated to keep your body working perfectly and improve your overall well-being.

Keep in mind that drinking more water is only a small part of your overall wellness strategy in the absence of calorie restriction and/or physical activity. Simply drinking water will not result in significant weight loss. As is always the case, a more comprehensive and long-term strategy is required for the best results.

Chapter 5: Breakfast Recipes That Are High in Protein and Low in Fat

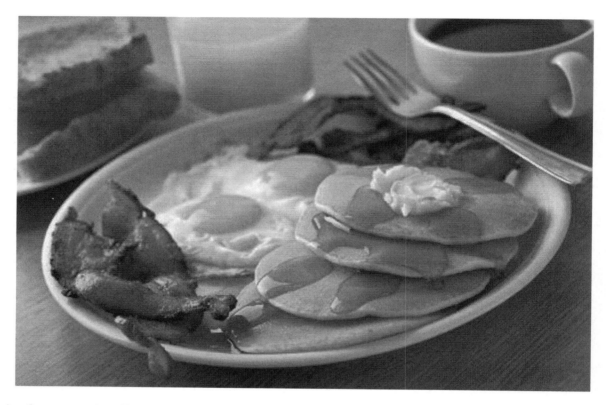

Calories from protein affect your brain, your appetite control center, so you are more satiated and satisfied.

1. Breakfast Loaded Pepper

Prep time: 10 mins

Cooking time: 30-40 mins

Servings: 1-2

Ingredients:

- 1 large-sized red bell pepper
- ½ C. canned black beans
- ½ C. thinly diced cherry tomatoes
- ½ tsp. chipotle sauce of your choice

- ½ C. parmesan cheese
- ¼ tsp. pink Himalayan salt
- Pinch of turmeric
- Pinch of black pepper
- 2 medium-sized eggs
- Garnishing of your choice

Directions:

1. Preheat the oven to 350°F. Cut the bell pepper half lengthwise and remove all the seeds and membranes.
2. Take a medium-sized bowl and combine cooked rice, tomatoes, beans, parmesan, salt, turmeric, and the chipotle sauce.
3. Divide the mixture among the two halves of the pepper equally. Take a small spoon and make an indention in the center of the pepper to add egg later.
4. Place the stuffed peppers into the oven and bake them for 20 minutes. Remove from oven and add one unbeaten egg in each created indention in the pepper. Bake again for 15 minutes and season with black pepper and garnishing of your choice.

Nutritional Values:

Calories: 450kcal

Sodium: 520mg

Fat: 2.1g

Carbohydrates: 120.7g

Cholesterol: 300.3 mg

Protein: 25.5g

2. Chia Pudding with Seasonal Fruit

Prep time: 20 mins

Cooking time: 0 mins

Serving: 1

Ingredients:

For Chia Pudding:

- 1 C. skimmed fat-free milk
- ½ C. chia seeds

For Seasonal Fruit:

- 1 Kiwi
- ½ Blood Orange
- 1 Valencia Orange
- 1 Passion Fruit
- ¼ C. Strawberries
- ¼ C. Blueberries

Instructions:

1. Soak chia seeds in a cup of fat-free milk, cover with plastic film and refrigerate overnight to get the best creaminess and thickness of the pudding.
2. Cut kiwi into slices and the rest of the fruit according to your liking. Take a flat plate and creatively layer the fruit onto it.
3. Take a spoon and scoop out the chia pudding from the bowl, top it onto the decorated fruit plate as desired, and dive into this yummy fruit chia pudding heaven.

Nutritional Values:

Calories: 458.65kcal

Sodium: 3mg

Fat: 2.6g

Carbohydrates: 120.7g

Cholesterol: 0mg

Protein: 27g

3. Protein Boost Breakfast Muffins

Prep time: 15 mins

Cooking time: 15 mins

Serving: 1

Ingredients:

- ½ C. gluten-free baking flour
- 1 ½ tbsp. protein powder (preferably vanilla)
- ¼ tsp. Baking powder
- ¼ fat-free Greek yogurt
- ½ tsp. unsweetened almond milk

For Cinnamon Sugar Coating:

- ¾ tsp. butter
- ½ tbsp. sugar substitute (sacral)
- ½ tsp. cinnamon

Instructions

1. Preheat the oven to 350°F and grease a ramekin with butter.
2. Take a medium-sized bowl and add flour, protein powder, and baking powder. Mix it well.
3. Gradually add Greek yogurt and almond milk while stirring gently. As soon as a dough consistency is formed, stop mixing.
4. Slightly wet your palms, divide the dough into 6 pieces, and roll it into a ball shape.
5. For the cinnamon sugar coating, melt butter in a bowl and combine sugar substitute and cinnamon in another separate bowl.
6. Roll the ball evenly in the butter and place it in the sugar-cinnamon mixture to coat it lightly. Repeat the same process for every dough ball.
7. Bake for 10 to 12 minutes until a toothpick inserted comes out clean.

Nutritional Values:

Calories: 340kcal

Fat: 3g

Carbohydrates: 60.7g

Protein: 25.5g

4. Berry-ola Yogurt Breakfast Bowl

Prep time: 15mins

Cooking time: 0 mins

Serving: 1

Ingredients:

- ½ C. sliced strawberries or any other berry fruit of your choice.
- ½ C. blueberries (Fresh)
- ½ tsp. substitute sugar
- 4–5 mint leaves
- 4 Oz. low-fat plain Greek yogurt
- ¼ c. granola
- 1 tbsp. protein powder (flavored)

Instructions:

1. Take a broad-mouthed wine glass and add half quantity of the fruit into it.
2. Take a blender and blend in the yogurt with the rest of the fruits in it. You can use a hand blender too. Do not over blend it. Make sure the strawberries and berries are a bit chunky.
3. Pour the blended mixture into the wine glass over the fruits. You can layer the fruits on the top, depending on your liking.
4. Mix the protein powder with yogurt and give it a quick whisk. Layer granola onto the yogurt in any way you want.
5. Enjoy a spoonful of this fruity yogurt heaven with granola crunch. The best super breakfast bowl that saves time too.

Nutritional Values:

Calories: 300kcal

Sodium: 100mg

Fat: 2.7g

Carbohydrates: 70g

Protein: 19.5g

5. Protein Pancakes

Prep time: 10 mins

Cooking time: 15 mins

Serving: 2

Ingredients:

- 40g Quaker instant Oats
- 1 medium-sized egg
- 1tbsp. fat-free milk
- Pint of cinnamon
- ½ large-sized banana
- Olive oil or any other flavorless oil for cooking
- Nut butter to serve
- ½ tbsp. baking powder
- 2 tbsp. protein powder

Instructions:

1. Take a large bowl and add banana, oats, eggs, cinnamon, milk, protein powder, and baking powder.
2. Mix all the ingredients until a batter consistency is formed. If you like, you can keep the banana a bit chunky too but make sure it is mixed well among the batter. If necessary, use a hand blender, or just whisk all the ingredients for 2 to 3 minutes.
3. Drizzle oil on a medium heat pan. Use a large pan so that 2 to 3 pancakes can be made at a time. Take a deep spoon and pour 2-3 spoonfuls of the batter in the pan with a space of 3 inches among each batter poured to allow space for spreading.
4. Cook for 1 to 2 minutes and allow it to form a solid shape. Once it is not gooey anymore, toss it upside down and cook the other side for another 1-2 minutes until a beautiful golden-brown color appears.

5. Immediately place it in a hot pot or a warm oven and repeat the process for the remaining batter. Once all cooked, layer the pancakes and serve in stacks. Spread some nut butter or serve it as a dip.

6. Enjoy the best protein-packed pancakes with a nutty flavor.

Nutritional Values:

Calories: 450kcal

Fat: 2.5g

Carbohydrates: 120.7g

Protein: 31g

6. The Best Scrambled Eggs

Prep time: 10mins

Cooking time: 15 mins

Serving: 1

Ingredients:

- 1 tbsp. + 1 tsp. olive oil
- 3 cherry tomatoes, halved
- 2 large eggs
- 2 tbsp. natural yogurt
- 5 leaves of basil, fresh, chopped
- 85g baby spinach (fully dried if it needs to be washed)
- ½ tsp. black pepper
- ¼ tsp. salt

Instructions:

1. Bring a large nonstick frying pan to medium heat and drizzle 1 tbsp. of coconut oil.

2. Add the halved cherry tomatoes (cut side down) and cook them for 2 to 3 minutes.

3. While the tomatoes are cooking, beat two eggs in a jug and add black pepper, salt, yogurt, chopped basil leaves, and 2 tbsp. of water. Mix all the ingredients.

4. Transfer the cooked tomatoes to a serving plate. Add spinach to the used pan and wilt it for a while.

5. Add another teaspoon of coconut oil, pour the beaten egg mixture into the pan, and cook it for half a minute with the baby spinach.

6. Cook until the eggs appear fluffy and set.

7. Transfer eggs into the serving plate and enjoy it with cooked tomatoes.

Nutritional Values:

Calories: 400kcal

Sodium: 0.6g

Fat: 2.8g

Carbohydrates: 10g

Protein: 25.5g

7. Choco Spinach Milk

Prep time: 5 mins

Cooking time: 0 mins

Serving: 1

Ingredients:

- 195 ml unsweetened soy milk
- 160g fat-free Greek yogurt
- 20g cooked quinoa
- 3 tbsp. cocoa powder
- ½ tsp. fresh vanilla beat extract
- ½ tsp. cinnamon
- 3 cubes of frozen spinach

Instructions:

1. Blend the ingredients in a blender or use a hand blender if available. Mix it well until a smooth chunky-free consistency is formed.

2. Pour in a glass and serve chilled.

Nutritional Values:

Calories: 280kcal

Sodium: 0.4g

Fat: 1.6g

Carbohydrates: 14g

Protein: 28g

8. Protein-Packed Breakfast Steak

Prep time: 20 mins

Cooking time: 20-30 mins

Serving: 1

Ingredients:

- 12ml extra virgin olive oil
- 3 cherry tomatoes, diced into half
- 2 turkey bacon strips
- 180g sirloin steak, fat trimmed
- 100g baby spinach
- 100g sliced mushrooms of your choice (canned)
- 1 medium-sized egg

Instructions:

1. Preheat the oven to 200°F. Take a pan and cover it with foil paper. Place half-cut cherry tomatoes, drizzle oil on top, and season well. Place pan in the oven and bake tomatoes for 5 minutes.

2. Add turkey bacon to the pan and cook it with tomatoes for 5 minutes or until it is cooked through. Turn the oven off and keep the pan inside so that the meal stays warm.

3. Take a frying pan and bring it on a high flame. Add the remaining extra oil into it and let the pan get hot.

4. Meanwhile, season the steak according to your taste and liking and when the pan gets very hot, cook the steak from each side for 4-5 minutes, altering the flame from medium to high and vice versa.

5. Once cooked, let sit for 1 minute and transfer it to a hot metal plate or a regular ceramic plate. In the same pan, set on a medium flame, add the mushrooms, and cook them until well sautéed. Move them to one side of a pan and now add spinach and cook it for a while in all those leftover steak juices. Once cooked, transfer it to the steak plate.

6. Meanwhile, bring a pan of water to boil and crack an egg into it. Poach the egg for 3-5 minutes until the yolk is runny and the white is cooked and set. Once cooked, lift it out with a strainer spoon and drain all the excess water.

7. Place the egg on top of the steak and all the other prepared meals on the side of the plate.

8. Serve hot.

Nutritional Values:

Calories: 686kcal

Sodium: 2.8g

Fat: 7g

Carbohydrates: 5g

Protein: 87g

9. Slow Cook Breakfast Beans

Prep time; 10 mins

Cooking time: 1h 40mins

Serving: 1

Ingredients:

- 1 tbsp. extra virgin olive oil
- 1 small sized onion, chopped
- 2 garlic cloves, chopped
- 1 tbsp. red wine vinegar or grape vinegar
- ½ tbsp. brown sugar, soft
- 100g pinto beans (canned)
- 100ml tomato puree (canned)
- 1 small bunch of coriander, finely chopped

- 1 large egg

Instructions:

1. Turn on the slow cooker if required first. Take a medium-sized frying pan, bring it to medium flame and drizzle olive oil.

2. Add onion and sauté it for 2-3 minutes until it turns brown, then add the chopped garlic and cook for another minute.

3. Add vinegar and brown sugar and stir it for 30-45 seconds until it gets bubbly. Pour the beans (rinsed and drained) and add the tomato puree. Stir for a while and season with black pepper

4. Transfer everything to the slow cooker and cook it for 5 hours until the beans are cooked through and thicken the tomato puree. If the puree seems thin, then increase the temperature and cook it on high heat for a while.

5. Meanwhile, fry an egg and place it on a serving plate.

6. Pour the cooked beans on the plate and enjoy it with an egg.

Nutritional Values:

Calories: 405kcal

Sodium: 0.39g

Fat: 2.6g

Carbohydrates: 21g

Protein: 12g

10. Overnight Oats

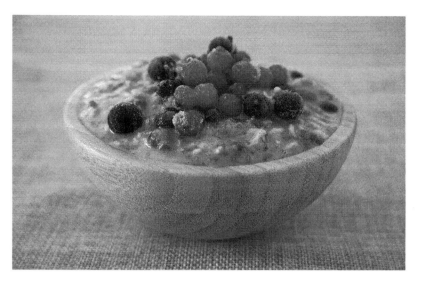

Prep time: Overnight

Cooking time: 0 mins

Serving: 1

Ingredients:

- 1 tsp. powdered matcha

- ½ C. oats, rolled

- 1 tbsp. chia seeds

- ½ C. fat-free milk

- ½ C. Greek yogurt, simple and low in fat

- ½ C. mango, pineapple, or kiwi, or a combination of the three

- 1 tbsp. unsweetened dried coconut flakes

Instructions:

1. To prepare the matcha paste, place it in a small bowl with 1 tablespoon of hot water and whisk until it becomes smooth and silky. (This helps break up any clumps and allows the taste to develop before mixing with the other ingredients).

2. Combine oats and chia seeds in a jar or container with a tight-fitting cover and shake well. Add the milk, yogurt, and matcha paste to a mixing bowl. Stir everything, cover, and place in the refrigerator overnight or

for up to 5 days. Before serving, stir in the mango, pineapple, or kiwi and top with the coconut flakes, then serve immediately.

Nutritional Values:

Calories: 430kcal

Sodium: 100mg

Fat: 4g

Carbohydrates: 59g

Protein: 26g

11. Fruity Protein Bowl

Prep time: 15 mins

Cooking time: 0 mins

Serving: 1

Ingredients:

- 1 large banana, frozen

- ½ C. almond milk

- 3 tbsp. protein powder

- 1 C. spinach

- Ice cubes as desired

For Toppings:

- Unsalted almond butter

- Roasted almonds

- Chia seeds of your choice

- Granola, low fat

- Strawberries, sliced

- Coconut flakes

Instructions:

1. Blend all ingredients in a high-powered blender until thick and creamy, except for the desired toppings. Almond milk and/or ice can be added as needed to get the appropriate consistency. You should consume the smoothie with a spoon since it should be thick enough.

2. Pour in a bowl and top with the remaining toppings.

Nutritional Values:

Calories: 300kcal

Fat: 4g

Carbohydrates: 50g

Protein: 20g

12. Blueberry Turkey Kebabs

Prep time: 10 mins

Cooking time: 10 mins

Serving: 1-2

Ingredients:

- ½ lb. lean ground turkey

- 1 garlic clove, crushed

- ½ tbsp. Maple syrup

- ½ tbsp. sage leaves, chopped

- ¼ tsp. Dried thyme leaves powder

- ¼ tsp. cumin

- ½ tsp. Ginger paste

- ¼ tsp. garam masala

- ¼ tsp. Cayenne pepper

- ½ tsp. pink salt

- Black pepper acc. to taste

- ½ C. fresh blueberries

- 1 tsp. olive oil

Instructions:

1. Mix all ingredients in a large bowl, except the blueberries and oil, with your hands until thoroughly incorporated. Blueberries should be added last and gently incorporated into the meat. Form into four equal-sized patties. Ensure that the blueberries are nestled into the meat; otherwise, they will pop out during the cooking process.

2. In a nonstick skillet, heat 1 teaspoon coconut oil over medium heat. Cook for about 5 minutes before flipping and cooking for an additional 4-5 minutes or until thoroughly done.

3. Pair two breakfast burgers with two fried eggs to create a platter. Drizzle a little amount of maple syrup over the sausage patties and serve! Serves four with two patties each.

Nutritional Values:

Calories: 350kcal

Fat: 4g

Carbohydrates: 5.9g

Protein: 22g

13. Besan Pancake

Prep time: 10 mins

Cooking time: 10 mins

Serving: 1

Ingredients:

- ¼ C. green onion, finely chopped

- ¼ C green pepper

- ½ C. chickpea flour or Besan

- ¼ tsp. pink salt

- ¼ tsp. black pepper

- ¼ tsp. baking powder

- A pinch of red pepper flakes (optional)

- ½ c. + 2 tbsp. water

Instructions:

1. Prep and put aside the veggies. Preheat a skillet 10 inches in diameter over medium heat.

2. Mix the chickpea flour, garlic powder, salt, pepper, baking powder, and optional red pepper flakes in a small bowl until combined.

3. Whisk in the water until no clumps remain. Mix it for about 15 seconds to infuse the batter with air bubbles. Vegetables, chopped, should be added at this point.

4. Spray the skillet generously with olive oil or another nonstick cooking spray after it is preheated (a drop of water should sizzle on the pan).

5. Pour the batter onto the pan and rapidly spread it out. Cook for about 5-6 minutes on one side or until a pancake flipper/spatula slides easily under the pancake and it is solid enough to flip without breaking.

6. Cook for a further 5 minutes, or until gently browned on the opposite side. Cook for an adequate amount of time since this pancake cooks much more slowly than standard pancakes.

7. Distribute evenly on a large platter and garnish with chosen toppings.

Nutritional Values:

Calories:: 306kcal

Fat: 2g

Carbohydrates: 25g

Protein: 25g

14. Heavenly Tempeh Sandwich

Prep time: 5 mins

Cooking time: 7 mins

Serving: 2

Ingredients:

- 3 tbsp. soy sauce
- 1 tbsp. maple syrup
- 1 tbsp. Grape vinegar
- ½ tsp. garlic paste
- 1 tsp. paprika powder
- Black pepper to taste
- 4 oz. tempeh, sliced
- 1 tbsp. olive oil
- 2 slices fat-free whole wheat bread
- ½ C. baby spinach
- Dressing of your choice

Instructions:

1. Whisk together the soy sauce, maple syrup, vinegar, garlic, paprika, and pepper in a small bowl.
2. Cut the tempeh in half thickness-wise using a sharp knife, creating two thin slabs. Slice each slab in half or thirds to create a total of 4-6 slabs.
3. Coat a big pan with olive oil and heat over moderately high heat. Cook the tempeh slabs in a uniform layer for approximately 3 minutes or until the bottoms are browned. Pour soy sauce mixture over tempeh and continue cooking for another minute or two, or until the sauce thickens and creates a coating on the tempeh.
4. Cook for about 3 more minutes, or until the tempeh slabs are browned on both sides, and the majority of the liquid has evaporated.
5. Spread any dressing on the bread and stuff the bread with tempeh slabs.

Nutritional Values:

Calories: 573kcal

Fat: 4g

Carbohydrates: 40g

Protein: 29g

Chapter 6: Lunch Recipes That Are High in Protein and Low in Fat

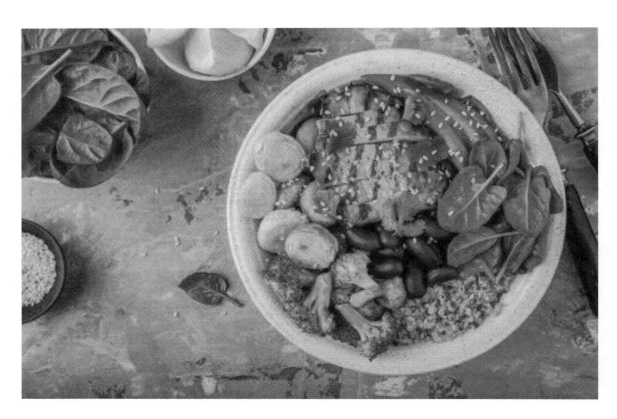

1. Tuna Kebabs

Prep time: 15 mins

Cooking time: 15 mins

Serving: 1-2

Ingredients:

- 6 Oz. canned tuna chunks
- ¼ C. fat-free mayo
- ¼ C. chopped onion
- 1 large egg
- ½ tbsp. dried parsley.

- ½ tsp. garlic powder
- ½ tsp. pink salt
- ¼ tsp. black pepper
- ½ tsp. cornflour

For the Lemon Sauce:

- ½ C. fat-free mayo
- 1 zested lemon
- 1 clove of garlic
- 1 squeezed lemon
- ½ tsp. salt
- ¼ tsp. black pepper

Instructions:

1. Drain water from the tuna and keep it aside to semi-dry. Take a medium-sized bowl and add onion and parsley.
2. Add tuna in the same bowl as onion and parsley and mix all three ingredients well. Make sure not to break tuna chunks.
3. Add egg, mayo, corn flour, salt, pepper, and garlic. Mix until thoroughly and evenly spread out on tuna.
4. When the mixture is ready, let it sit for 5 to 10 mins. Make the shape of your choice using a shaping tool or hand. Drizzle oil in a nonstick pan and cook the kebabs on medium flame until light golden brown. Toss on the sides and make sure to cook each side for more than 5 to 10 minutes on medium heat.
5. Add mayo, garlic paste, lemon zest, salt, pepper, and squeezed lemon in a small bowl. Give it a quick whisk and serve with hot tuna kebabs as a dip.

Nutritional Values:

Calories: 350kcal

Fat: 3.2g

Carbohydrates: 8g

Protein: 40g

2. Lentil Salad with Vegetable

Prep Time: 15 mins

Cooking time: 20 mins

Serving: 1

Ingredients:

- 100g lentils (you may choose any lentils), rinsed and drained

- ¼ C. red-onion, chopped

- ¼ C. red bell pepper, chopped

- ¼ C. cucumber, chopped

- 3 cherry tomatoes, halved

- 1 bunch of fresh parsley, chopped

- ½ tbsp. lemon juice

- 2 tbsp. extra virgin olive oil

- 1 tsp. pink-salt

- Pint of Black-pepper

Instructions:

1. Soak lentils in water for 30 to 40 minutes to soften them up slightly.

2. Bring a pan of water to boil and add in the lentils. Boil until the lentils are cooked through and eatable.

3. Take a mixing bowl and add all the chopped vegetables and lemon juice. Give it a light mix, and add oil, salt, and black pepper.

4. Add the boiled lentils to the vegetables and mix the ingredients well together.

5. Serve in a dish and enjoy the freshness of this meal.

Nutritional Values:

Calories: 300kcal

Fat: 2.3g

Carbohydrates: 30g

Protein: 18g

Sodium: 49mg

3. Honey Mustard Baked Chicken

Prep time: 20 mins

Cooking time: 20 mins

Serving: 2

Ingredients:

- 1 tbsp. Pink salt.

- 2 tsp. paprika powder

- 1 tsp. sundried onion powder

- 1 tsp. garlic powder

- 1 tbsp. honey

- 1 C. low-fat buttermilk

- 1 ½ lb. chicken skinless, boneless breasts cut into ¼ inch size strips (this will make around 7 to 8 strips) chicken tenderloins

- 2 C. crispy breadcrumbs

- 2 tbsp. Extra virgin olive oil.

- 2 egg whites, beaten.

- 1 tbsp. mustard sauce

- ½ C. nonfat Greek yogurt

Instructions:

1. Take a large empty bowl and combine ½ tbsp. Pink salt, 1tsp. Paprika, ½ tsp. Onion powder, and ½ tsp. Garlic powder. Add ½ tbsp. Honey and buttermilk and mix all the ingredients until evenly combined.

2. Add the chicken tender strips to the batter and coat each side evenly. Let it sit for not more than 10 minutes, or it may become extra salty.

3. Take a large 1-inch-deep pan. Combine breadcrumbs and dry seasonings like paprika, garlic powder, onion powder, and salt. Mix it well together so that the spices are evenly distributed.

4. In another clean dish, add the egg whites and mustard sauce and whisk the two ingredients together

5. Preheat oven to 350°F. Place a baking pan covered with foil and a wire rack on top. The rack must be brushed or sprayed with cooking oil.

6. Now place the mixtures prepared side by side, including the breadcrumbs mixture, egg whites' mixture, and marinated chicken.

7. Take one well-coated strip in the seasoning and add it to the egg white mixture. Toss and turn it, so no side remains dry. Once it is wet, add it to the breadcrumbs mixture and allow a thin crumbs coating. Once done, place it on the baking sheet. Repeat the same process for the other strips.

8. Bake the chicken for 15 to 20 minutes until golden brown

9. For the dip, stir the ingredients of the dip, including mustard sauce, Greek yogurt, salt, and a tsp. of honey. Mix well and serve with tender strips.

Nutritional Values:

Calories: 460kcal

Fat: 2.5g

Carbohydrates: 35g

Protein: 35g

Cholesterol: 1g

Sodium: 104mg

4. Kale Wraps with Turkey

Prep time: 10 mins

Cooking time: 10 mins

Serving: 2

Ingredients:

- 1 tbsp. cranberry sauce

- 1 tsp. mustard sauce

- 3 medium-sized kale leaves

- 5 oz. turkey, sliced

- 1 red onion, chopped

- 1 medium-sized pear, Sliced

Instructions:

1. Mix cranberry sauce and mustard sauce in a bowl and then spread a layer of it on the kale leaves as a base sauce

2. Place a slice of turkey, onion according to your taste, and 2 slices of pear into the wrap, layering the ingredients.

3. Wrap and fold the kale leaves once the stuffing is complete and serve with a dip of your choice.

Nutritional Values:

Calories: 395kcal

Fat: 2.1g

Carbohydrates: 40g

Protein: 27g

5. Turkey Kofta

Prep time: 15 mins

Cooking time: 30 mins

Serving: 2

Ingredients:

- 10 Oz. minced turkey (white meat)

- 1-oz fresh or frozen spinach

- ¼ C. Quaker instant oats

- 2 egg whites

- 1 celery stick

- 2 cloves of garlic

- ½ large green bell pepper (membrane and seeds removed)

- ½ medium-sized red onion

- ½ C. parsley (fresh)

- ½ tsp. cumin seeds

- 1 tsp. mustard powder

- 1 tsp. dry thyme

- ½ tsp. turmeric powder

- ½ tsp. chipotle-pepper

- ¼ tsp. pink Himalayan salt

- Pint of black pepper

Instructions:

1. Preheat the oven to 350°F.

2. Finely chop garlic, onion, and celery (you may also use a food-processor gadget to speed up the chopping process) and shift into a mixing bowl.

3. Add minced turkey (white meat), 2 egg whites, oats, and spices to the container and mix until all the ingredients are combined well. Make sure that there are no lumps of oats in the mixture.

4. Chop fresh or frozen spinach, green peppers, and parsley and transfer all of this to the mixing bowl.

5. Mix and combine the ingredients well altogether completely.

6. Line a baking sheet with butter paper.

7. Once again, mix the ingredients well and refrigerate the mixture for 10 to 15 minutes.

8. Make meatballs out of the mixture in whatever size you want. Lay the meatballs out on a baking sheet.

9. Bake for 25 minutes until the meatballs are cooked through or insert a fork and check the softness of the meat.

10. Serve these balls with a drizzle of lemon juice.

Nutritional Values:

Calories: 300kcal

Fat: 2.5g

Carbohydrates: 12g

Protein: 30g

6. Shrimp & Black Bean Salad

Prep time: 10 mins

Cooking time 2 mins

Serving: 2

Ingredients:

- 2-tbsp. Organic grape vinegar

- 1 tbsp. lime juice

- 1 tsp. extra virgin olive oil

- ½ tsp. red chili flakes

- Pint of pink salt

- ½ C. brown rice

- 1 C. corn kernels (Canned)

- 100g canned black beans (rinsed and drained)

- 2 Oz. cooked shrimps (cut into bite-size pieces)

- 1 medium-sized tomato (bite-sized chunks)

- 1 small branch of scallion, chopped

- 3 tbsp. chopped fresh cilantro (optional)

Instructions:

1. Take a medium-sized mixing bowl and add vinegar, oil, lime juice, salt, and chili flakes.

2. Add boiled rice, black beans, corn, tomato, shrimps, cilantro (optional), and scallions. Mix all the ingredients well together until an evenly combined mixture is formed.

3. Stir-fry all the ingredients lightly in a pan on high heat to get the best taste and texture of the meal.

4. Check the taste and adjust seasoning (if needed, add more lime juice, vinegar, chili powder, and salt according to taste).

5. Serve fresh, or it can be stored in the refrigerator for up to 2 days.

Nutritional Values:

Calories: 334kcal

Fat: 2.6g

Carbohydrates: 33g

Protein: 20g

7. Lemon-Pepper Chicken Breasts

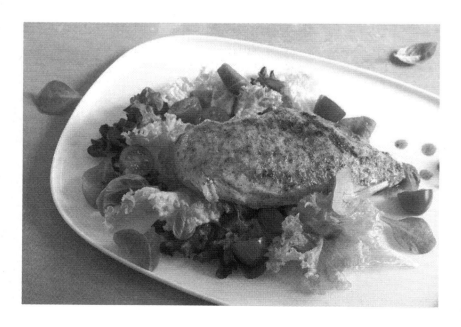

Prep time: 5 mins

Cooking time: 15 mins

Serving: 2

Ingredients:

- 1 (11 Oz.) chicken breast, sliced in half through the thickness.

- 1 tbsp. almond flour

- 1 tsp. dried Italian powder

- 1 tsp. Black pepper

- ¾ tsp. Pink salt

- ½ tsp. garlic powder

- 1 tbsp. extra virgin olive oil

- 2 tsp. Nonfat butter from the brand "I can't believe it's not butter".

- 1 ½ tbsp. fresh lemon juice,

- 1 tsp. lemon zest

- 1 tbsp. chopped parsley (fresh)

Instructions

1. Take a medium-sized mixing bowl and put together flour, Italian seasoning, salt, garlic powder, and pepper to taste.

2. Mix all the dry ingredients well and marinate the chicken breasts with the spices over both sides of the chicken.

3. Melt the nonfat butter into a nonstick frying pan over medium heat. Cook the marinated chicken breasts until a golden-brown color appears.

4. Once the chicken is nearly tender, add olive oil and cook for another 2 to 3 minutes until the chicken becomes tender and juicy. Make sure not to over-dry the chicken.

5. Once cooked completely, turn off the flame and drizzle lemon juice on top of the chicken along with the lemon zest

6. Garnish with freshly cut parsley and serve hot or warm.

Nutritional Values:

Calories: 360kcal

Fat: 2g

Carbohydrates: 1g

Protein: 33g

8. Vegan Sweet Potato Soup Curry

Prep time: 10 mins

Cooking time: 40 mins

Serving: 2

Ingredients:

*   1 large-sized green-bell pepper finely chopped

*   400 ml. tomato puree

*   1 medium-sized sweet potato, chunked

*   ½ medium sized-onion, chopped

*   2 cloves of garlic, crushed

*   70g canned kidney beans, rinsed and dried

*   1 tsp. Pink salt

*   ½ tsp. black pepper

*   1 tsp. cumin seeds

*   1 tbsp. chicken powder

*   1 tbsp. corn flour or any other thickening agent

- 1 tsp. Paprika powder

- ½ tsp. Chili powder

- ½ tsp. dried oregano

- Avocado and cilantro for garnishing

- 600ml. water

- 1tbsp. olive oil

Instructions

1. Pour water into a medium-sized deep pan and bring it to low flame.

2. Add in all the ingredients mentioned above except the garnishing and corn flour. Stir well for 2 to 3 minutes until everything is combined well.

3. Cover the pot with the lid for 20 minutes to create steam. This will help with cooking the potatoes fast.

4. Once the soup comes to a boil, remove the lid and stir gently for 1-2 minutes. Alter the flame from low to medium and allow it to cook for another 10 minutes until the potatoes are cooked through, and the consistency gets thicker.

5. Add the corn flour and stir well to avoid any flour lumps immediately.

6. Once everything is cooked through and softened, check for the spices and add more salt if needed.

7. Garnish with avocado and cilantro and serve hot.

Nutritional Values:

Calories: 420kcal

Fat: 2.22g

Carbohydrates: 89g

Protein: 20g

9. Puy Lentils Burger

Prep time: 5 mins

Cooking time: 20 mins

Serving: 2

Ingredients:

- ¼ C. green Puy lentils

- ½ tsp. pink salt

- 1 tbsp. extra virgin olive oil

- ½ small onion, diced

- ½ green bell pepper, diced

- 2 cloves of garlic (paste)

- 1 Oz. green chiles, chopped

- 200ml. tomato puree

- 2 tbsp. organic ketchup

- ½ tbsp. mustard sauce

- ½ tbsp. vegan Worcestershire sauce

- ¼ tbsp. chili powder

- 2 tbsp. organic grape vinegar

- Pint of black pepper

- 2 thin slices of turkey (cooked)

- 2 whole-wheat hamburger buns, whole

- 2 medium-sized kale leaves

- Avocado, for serving

Instructions:

1. Bring the lentils to boil in a saucepan and cover the lid to speed up the process. Add salt and simmer the lentils for 1-2 minutes over low heat. Once the lentils are cooked and tender, for roughly 30 minutes, remove from flame and drain the water.

2. Take a large nonstick frying pan and bring it over medium heat. Add the onion and bell pepper and sauté until the onions appear transparent and the bell peppers appear slightly tender and crispy.

3. Add in garlic paste and chiles and cook for 1 minute. Once cooked, pour in the tomato puree and mix it quickly.

4. Gradually add ketchup, mustard sauce, all the mentioned spices, grape vinegar, and Worcestershire sauce. Mix all the ingredients well together on a medium flame and gently stir for 2-3 minutes until the sauce comes to a sizzling point.

5. Add in ¼ C of water and cook for another 10 minutes. Keep cooking until the desired thickness of the sauce is created.

6. Turn the flame off once the sauce is ready, and add the boiled lentils. Mix everything gently and cover the pan with the lid to keep it warm.

7. Meanwhile, lightly toast the hamburger buns and spread butter on the inner sides. Place one kale leaf on the hamburger bun, layering the lentils mixture prepared on top. You can keep the quantity as desired. Layer a slice of turkey on top of the lentils and finally place the upper bun on it. Repeat the same layering process for the second hamburger.

8. Serve warm and serve avocados as a side meal along with it.

Nutritional Values:

Calories: 400kcal

Fat: 3g

Carbohydrates: 69g

Protein: 20g

10. Spinach with Apple Sauce Chicken

Prep time: 10 mins

Cooking time: 20 mins

Serving: 2

Ingredients:

- ¼ C. apple sauce

- 1 tbsp. low-sodium soya sauce

- 2 tsp. Fresh thyme

- ½ tsp. Lemon zest

- ½ tsp. ginger paste

- 4 oz. (skin-less and bone-less), chicken breast (cut in halves)

- ½ tbsp. pink salt

- Black pepper to taste

- 1 tbsp. olive oil

- 1 medium apple, chopped

- Half onion, chopped

- 1 tsp. garlic paste

- 3 C. spinach, leaves chopped

Instructions:

1. Combine the apple sauce, thyme, soy sauce, lemon peel, and ginger in a small microwave-safe container. Microwave for 60 seconds, or until jelly is completely melted, and save 2 tablespoons of the apple glaze.
2. Generously season chicken breasts with salt and pepper.
3. Arrange chicken on cooled broiler pan frame and broil for 15 minutes, turning once and brushing chicken with remaining glaze during the final 3 minutes of broiling.
4. Spray the nonstick pan with cooking oil if it has not been warmed.
5. Preheat over a medium flame. Add the apple, garlic, and onion to a hot pan and cook for 2 minutes, stirring constantly.
6. Increase the heat to high and add the reserved glaze, stirring constantly.
7. Toss in the spinach and heat until barely done.
8. Evenly divide spinach mixture across two dinner plates and top with chicken slides.

Nutritional Values:

Calories: 450kcal

Fat: 3.2g

Carbohydrates: 41 g

Protein: 25g

11. White-Fish with Stew

Prep time: 20 mins

Cooking time: 1 h 10 mins

Serving: 1

Ingredients:

- 1tbs extra-virgin olive oil

- ½ onion, diced

- 1 tbsp. garlic paste

- ½ tsp. dried oregano

- ½ tsp. pink salt

- Black pepper to taste

- 1 C. water

- 1 medium-sized potato, cubes

- Codfish single serving or quantity of your choice

- 1 tbsp. lemon juice

Instructions:

1. Turn up the heat and add the oregano, garlic, salt, onion, and pepper to a pan.

2. Once the onion is soft, add some water and bring to a boil.

3. Reduce the heat from high to low, then cover and boil for another 30 minutes.

4. Add potatoes and continue to boil, covered, for an additional 15 minutes. With the assistance of a slotted spoon, transfer the potatoes to the container.

5. Incorporate the codfish into the gravy sauce. At the very least, the fish should be completely submerged in liquid (if needed, add some more water in a pan).

6. Place the potatoes in the saucepan and secure the top.

7. Boil until the codfish has changed color and the potatoes are tender.

8. Before serving, squeeze lemon juice over the stew.

Nutritional Values:

Calories: 300kcal

Fat: 2.9g

Carbohydrates: 26g

Protein: 18g

Sodium: 512mg

12. Sprouts Salad

Prep time: 5 Mins

Cooking time: 15 mins

Serving: 2

Ingredients:

- 2 c. sprouted moong beans

- 1 medium-sized onion, finely chopped

- 1 medium-size tomato, finely chopped

- 1 green chili, finely chopped, optional

- ¼ tsp. red chili, powder

- 1 tsp. lemon juice, or as required

- 1 boiled sweet potato, finely chopped

- A few coriander leaves for garnishing

- A few lemon slices for garnishing

- Pink salt, as required

Instructions:

1. To begin, steam or boil sprouts until they are thoroughly cooked. Then drain the cooked sprouts to eliminate any remaining liquid.

2. In a large container, combine two cups of steamed (or boiling) moong sprouts. Additionally, add finely chopped onion and tomatoes.

3. Stir in 1 finely chopped green chili and 1 cooked potato (optional).

4. Add the red chili and combine well.

5. Season with salt and drizzle lemon juice (or as required).

6. Combine well and garnish with coriander leaves and lemon zest.

Nutritional Values:

Calories: 230kcal

Fat: 1g

Carbohydrates: 20g

Protein: 15g

13. Low-Fat Spaghetti Squash

Prep time: 5 mins

Cooking time: 30 mins

Serving: 2

Ingredients:

For Spaghetti Squash:

- 1 small baked spaghetti squash
- 2 C. broccoli, steamed

For the Sauce:

- 3 c. (275 g) fresh spinach
- ¼ C soft tofu
- 1 C fresh basil leaves
- 1 tsp. nutritional yeast
- 3 cloves garlic
- ¼ tsp. pink Himalayan salt
- 1 tbsp. lemon juice

Instructions:

1. Cut the squash into half and place it on a baking ban. Use a spoon to clear out the gunky part of the quash and the uppermost thin layer for better taste.
2. Preheat the oven to 350°F and bake squash for 20-30 minutes.
3. Once cooked, peel the strands of the squash with the help of a fork to create the shape of spaghetti.
4. For the sauce, add all the sauce ingredients into a blender and mix until it remains a little bit chunky.
5. Add steamed broccoli to the cooked squash and drizzle the sauce over it, or you can also use the sauce as a dip.

Nutritional Values:

Calories: 309kcal

Fat: 3g

Carbohydrates: 20g

Protein: 18g

14. Cream of Chickpea Soup

Prep time: 20 mins

Cooking time: 1 h 30 mins

Serving: 2

Ingredients:

- 1 tsp. olive oil
- ¼ onion, chopped
- 1 tsp. garlic paste
- 1 celery stick, chopped
- 1 small potato, thinly diced
- 2 C. chickpeas
- ½ can tomato purée
- 3 C. water
- 1 tsp. fresh parsley
- ½ tsp. dried basil
- ½ tsp. dried oregano
- ½ tsp. salt or as needed
- Red chili flakes to taste
- 1 C. whole wheat pasta

Instructions:

1. In a large saucepan, combine olive oil, chopped onion, garlic, and celery; sauté for 2 minutes over low/medium heat, or until clear.
2. Add the potatoes, chickpeas, tomatoes, water, and spices and cook over low/medium heat until the potatoes are cooked and the sauce has thickened (approximately 60 minutes).
3. Cook the pasta until al dente for the last 15 minutes, then drain thoroughly.
4. Half of the prepared soup should be blended until smooth before returning to the saucepan with the pasta and heating until hot. If preferred, garnish with freshly grated parmesan cheese. Enjoy!

Nutritional Values:

Calories: 307kcal

Fat: 3.4g

Carbohydrates: 40g

Protein: 27g

Chapter 7: Dinner Recipes That Are High in Protein and Low in Fat

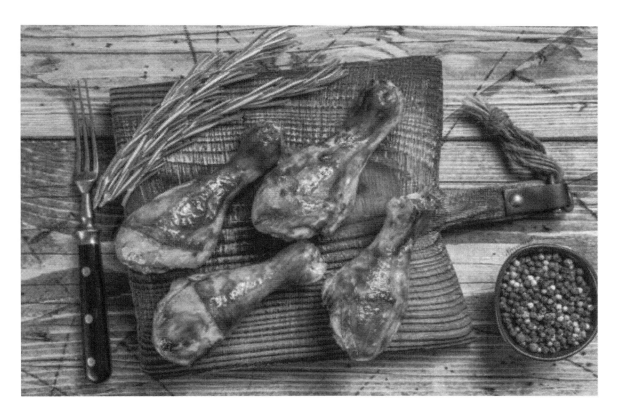

1. Red Lentil Soup

Prep time: 15 mins

Cooking time: 40 mins

Serving: 2

Ingredients:

- 1 Liter vegetable or chicken stock
- 75g red lentils
- 8 Oz. water
- 3 carrots, chopped
- 1 medium leek, sliced (about 150g)

- Chopped parsley
- ½ tsp. salt

Instructions:

1. Soak the lentils in water for 15 minutes in a medium bowl as it is a good tip for softening them up before cooking. Take a medium-sized cooking pot, add stock of your choice, and bring it to heat on a medium flame.

2. Add lentils to the stock and bring the stock to boil. Allow the lentils to soften for a few minutes.

3. Add carrots, salt, and leek and simmer for 15 minutes. Cover with the lid and cook it on low heat for 30 minutes until the lentils are cooked properly.

4. Garnish with freshly chopped parsley or any other seasoning of your choice and serve hot.

Nutritional Values:

Calories: 302kcal

Fat: 3g

Carbohydrates: 33g

Protein: 17g

2. Shrimp and Corn Pasta

Prep time: 5 mins

Cooking time: 30 mins

Serving: 2

Ingredients:

- 4 Oz. whole wheat pasta of any shape
- ½ lb. peeled raw shrimp
- 2 C. chopped spinach
- ½ C. cooked corn
- ½ C. frozen cooked peas
- 1 small onion
- 2 cloves of garlic, chopped

- 2 tbsp. tomato paste
- 1 tsp. paprika powder
- ¼ tsp. red saffron
- ¾ tsp. salt
- 2 C. water
- 2 tbsp. fresh parsley for garnishing

Instructions:

1. Combine all the above-listed ingredients in a large cooking pot except parsley.

2. Add in the two cups of water and stir evenly for 5 minutes on medium heat. Bring it to boil on a high heat eventually. Stir for another ten to fifteen minutes frequently until the pasta is cooked and the water has almost dried.

3. When the water has evaporated completely, remove the pot from heat and let it sit aside for 5 minutes, toss and mix gently and sprinkle some fresh cut parsley on top for garnish.

Nutritional Values:

Calories: 320kcal

Fat: 2g

Carbohydrates: 49g

Protein: 26g

3. Barbequed Chicken

Prep time: 10 mins

Cooking time: 30 mins

Serving: 2

Ingredients:

- 4 tbsp. fresh tomato paste
- 1 tsp. ketchup
- 1 tsp. Worcestershire sauce
- 4 tsp. Organic grape vinegar

- ¾ tsp. Cayenne pepper
- ½ tsp. Black pepper
- ¼ tsp. onion powder
- 2 cloves of garlic, paste form
- ⅛ tsp. garlic paste
- 1lb. chicken (breasts)

Instructions:

1. Combine all ingredients in a saucepan except chicken and mix well for 5 minutes on a low flame.
2. Wash chicken and let it dry for a while or dry it with tissue to save time. Place the chicken on a foil-wrapped baking sheet and brush the mixture on both sides of the chicken.
3. Heat the oven to 350°F and let the chicken grab all the flavors in the meantime. Place the chicken into the oven and bake it for 15 to 20 minutes until its fully cooked
4. Season with lemon or lime and serve hot.

Nutritional Values:

Calories: 420kcal

Fat: 3.2g

Carbohydrates: 7g

Protein: 25g

Sodium: 199g

4. Turkey Patties

Prep time: 5 mins

Cooking time: 10 mins

Serving: 2

Ingredients:

- ½ lb. turkey, minced
- 1 C. zucchini, finely chopped

- 1 tsp. garlic paste

- 1 tsp. cumin seeds, crushed

- Salt as per taste

- Black pepper as per taste

Instructions:

1. In a large bowl, combine minced lean turkey, zucchini, grated garlic, crushed cumin, and salt & pepper with the use of a hand-mixer.

2. Make three big turkey patties about the size of a medium hand.

3. Preheat a nonstick skillet/frypan over a low-medium heat setting. Turkey patties should be cooked over low and steady heat to ensure they are completely done.

4. Add about 1 tbsp. Oil to the pan and stir vigorously. Cook two patties in a pan for 5 minutes on each side, rotating halfway through. Repeat with the remainder of the oil and burger patties.

5. Take pleasure in this easy and delicious recipe.

Nutritional Values:

Calories: 301kcal

Fat: 1.8g

Carbohydrates: 1g

Protein: 18g

Sodium: 199g

5. Air Fryer Tofu Wrap

Prep time: 5 mins

Cooking time: 20 mins

Serving: 2

Ingredients:

- 14 oz. or 1 block extra firm tofu

- 2 tsp. Soy Sauce

- 1 tbsp. Sesame-Oil

- 1- tbsp. rice-vinegar

- 1- tsp. Sriracha-sauce (optional)

- 2 large iceberg lettuce leaves

- ½ red bell-pepper (deseeded and sliced)

- ½ C. red cabbage

- 2 cherry tomatoes, halved

- Sauce/dressing of your choice

Instructions:

1. Slice tofu into bite-sized cubes and set aside for a while.

2. Combine sesame oil, soy sauce, rice vinegar, and Sriracha sauce (optional).

3. Add tofu chunks and stir until evenly coated; set aside for approximately 20 minutes.

4. Preheat the air fryer to 375°F. Cook for 12 minutes, tossing tofu several times while cooking to ensure equal cooking.

5. Take the tofu out of the air fryer and let it cool down a bit.

6. Distribute iceberg lettuce on a plate and top with as much of each vegetable as desired, followed with Air Fried Tofu. Serve with a generous spoonful of sauce, as desired.

7. Fold the iceberg leaf and wrap the stuffing. Take pleasure in your delectable tofu wrap!

Nutritional Values:

Calories: 830kcal

Fat: 1.3g

Carbohydrates: 4g

Protein: 16g

Sodium: 63mg

6. Ginger Chicken Korean Style Bowl

Prep time: 10 mins

Cooking Time: 2 hrs. 25 mins

Serving: 2

Ingredients:

- ½ lb. chicken boneless, bite-sized chunks

- 1 medium-sized carrot, chopped

- 1 tsp. soy sauce

- 1 tsp. rice vinegar

- 1 tsp. ginger paste

- Black pepper to taste

- 6 oz. chicken or veggie stock.

- ½ C. water

- 1 oz. rice noodle

- 3 oz. pea pods, frozen and cut

Instructions:

1. Combine chicken, carrots, soy sauce, ginger, pepper, and vinegar in a cutlery cooker.

2. In a pressure cooker, combine chicken broth and water.

3. Cover the cooker and cook on high heat for 2 hours and 15 minutes. Add the noodles and pea pods into the cooker once the broth is ready.

4. Cover once again and continue cooking for an additional 5 minutes, or until noodles are tender.

5. Serve alongside soy sauce.

Nutritional Values:

Calories: 327kcal

Fat: 2.8g

Carbohydrates: 3g

Protein: 15g

Sodium: 78mg

7. Pork and Mushroom Gravy

Prep time: 10 mins

Cooking time: 45 mins

Serving: 2

Ingredients:

- 1 lb. pork, slice as desired

- Cooking oil spray

- 7 oz. fresh mushrooms

- ½ C. low sodium beef broth

- 2 tbsp. onion, chopped

- 1 tsp. Fresh rosemary

- ¼ tsp. Salt

- ¼ tsp. crushed black-pepper

- 1 tbsp. chickpea flour

- 1- tbsp. water

- 1- tbsp. fresh parsley

Instructions:

1. Remove the fat from pork meat.

2. Coat a big frying pan with nonstick cooking spray. Heat/flame frypan on medium heat.

3. Cook for 8 minutes or until the meat is browned. Turn the meat over and continue cooking for 5 minutes more, covered.

4. Combine mushrooms, broth, onion, wine/low sodium beef broth, and rosemary in a medium bowl. When it comes to a boil, turn off the heat. Continue simmering for 10 minutes.

5. Season the meat with salt and pepper.

6. Transfer meat to cutting board, cover, and set aside for 11 minutes.

7. In a small container, combine flour and water until smooth. Add broth mixture and heat, constantly stirring, until thick and bubbly.

8. To serve, cut meat slantwise into bits. Split the meat among serving plates and spoon the gravy over the meat, garnishing with parsley.

9. Take pleasure in your meal.

Nutritional Values:

Calories: 389kcal

Fat: 2.5g

Carbohydrates: 6.1g

Protein: 26.2g

Sodium: 30mg

8. Black Lentil Soup

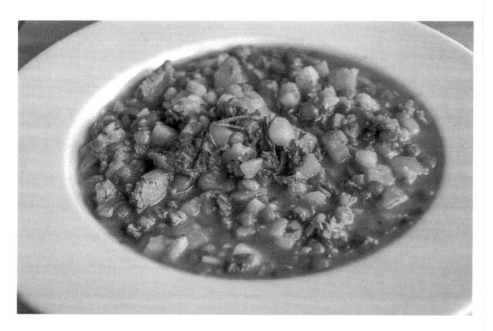

Prep time: 10 mins

Cooking time: 1 h 40 mins

Servings: 1

Ingredients:

- 1 C. black-eyed peas

- 2- tbsp. olive oil

- ½ diced yellow onion

- ½ large carrot, chopped

- 2 celery sticks, chopped

- 1 tsp. Garlic paste

- ½ tsp. paprika powder

- 1 tsp. Thyme and basil powder

- ½ tsp. onion powder

- 1 tsp. red chili flakes

- ½ tomato, paste form

- ½ C. green beans

- 3 C. veggie broth

- Salt and pepper to taste

Instructions:

1. Preheat oven to 350°F. Heat oil in a medium saucepan over medium heat. Add onion, carrots, and celery and cook for 7–10 minutes.

2. Cook garlic, smoked paprika, basil, thyme, oregano, and garlic-onion powder for approximately 2 minutes, or until aromatic.

3. Combine the Black-eyed peas, tomato, and vegetable broth in a saucepan. Bring to a boil, cover, turn to low heat, and simmer for 20 minutes (for canned) or until beans are cooked.

4. Stir in collard greens 5–10 minutes before the soup is finished.

5. Season with salt and pepper to taste. Squeeze a lemon over the serving dish. It is very delectable in flavor, nutrient-dense, and low in calories (also low in fat).

Nutritional Values:

Calories: 349kcal

Fat: 2.85g

Carbohydrates: 15g

Protein: 26g

Sodium: 56mg

9. Roasted Asparagus with Potato and Chicken

Prep time: 15 mins

Cooking time: 1 hr.

Servings: 2

Ingredients:

- 1 lb. red potatoes, cubes

- 1 C chicken chunks

- 2 tbsp. extra-virgin olive oil

- 2 tsp. garlic paste

- Rosemary and thyme as needed

- 1 tsp. pink salt

- 1 bunch fresh asparagus; 1-inch pieces

- grounded black-pepper for taste

Instructions:

1. Preheat oven to 420°F.

2. Toss red potatoes in a large baking dish with 1 tablespoon garlic, olive oil, rosemary, kosher salt, and thyme. Aluminum foil may be used to cover the dish.

3. Bake in a preheated oven for 21 minutes.

4. Combine asparagus and remaining salt and olive oil in a large mixing bowl. Increase the oven temperature to 445°F.

5. Remove aluminum foil and continue cooking for an additional 6 to 11 minutes, or until potatoes are lightly browned and soften. To serve, season with pepper. It is quite delectable in terms of flavor due to its simplicity and use of fewer ingredients.

6. Pair it with a simple roasted chicken breast marinated in your favorite sauce. Typically, marination of black pepper, turmeric, and salt complements the meal.

Nutritional Values:

Calories: 378kcal

Fat: 2.85g

Carbohydrates: 23g

Protein: 15g

Sodium: 576mg

10. Tomato Pasta with Basil

Prep time: 10 mins

Cooking time: 20 mins

Servings: 2

Ingredients:

- 8 oz. banza protein pasta uncooked spaghetti

- 2 C tomato paste, fresh

- 1 chopped tomato

- ½ C. basil leaves powder

- 1 tsp. garlic paste

- 1 tbsp. Olive oil plus 1 tsp. mustard oil

- Black pepper to taste

- 1 tbsp. lemon juice

- 1 oz. cottage cheese

Instructions:

1. Bring a medium-sized saucepan of lightly salted water to a boil. Boil the pasta for 8 to 10 minutes in a separate pot, then drain the water.

2. In a blender, mix chopped tomato (fresh tomatoes), garlic, basil, olive oil, and pepper until chunky, scraping down the sides as needed.

3. Gently toss the cooked tomato mixture and pasta into a separate container until well combined.

4. Before serving, drizzle lemon juice over the spaghetti and sprinkle with cottage cheese or chevre. This dish is quite easy to prepare with a limited amount of ingredients. Because all of the ingredients are fresh, the scent is enticing.

Nutritional Values:

Calories: 270kcal

Fat: 2.8g

Carbohydrates: 46g

Protein: 27g

Sodium: 246mg

11. Black-Beans with Brown Rice

Prep time: 10 mins

Cooking time: 30 mins

Serving: 2

Ingredients:

- 1 tsp. extra virgin olive oil

- ½ onion, chopped

- 2 cloves of garlic, minced

- 1 C. uncooked brown rice

- 1 ½ C low sodium/low-fat vegetable broth

- 1 tsp. crushed cumin

- ¼ tsp. cayenne pepper

- 1 C. tinned black beans (drained the liquid)

Instructions:

1. Heat the oil in a large stockpot over medium-high heat until shimmering.

2. Add onion and garlic and cook for 4 to 5 minutes until golden brown. Put the rice in the pan and cook for 2 to 3 minutes on medium heat. Make sure that you soak the rice in hot water for 10 to 15 minutes before to soften up the texture.

3. Fill everything with vegetable broth, bring it to a boil, cover it, reduce the heat to low, simmer for 20 minutes, and add spices and black beans to taste.

4. Add in lemon juice according to taste. Serve hot.

Nutritional Values:

Calories: 200kcal

Fat: 0.8g

Carbohydrates: 46g

Protein: 9g

Sodium: 266mg

12. Quorn Rice Bowl

Prep time: 5 mins

Cooking time: 20 mins

Serving: 3

Ingredients:

- 1 tsp. chili powder

- 1 tsp. Cumin powder

- ½ tsp. Salt

- ½ tsp. Garlic powder

- ¼ tsp. paprika, smoked

- Black pepper to taste

- 1 tbsp. olive oil or any other oil of your choice

- 1 lb. chicken tenders

- ½ onion, chopped

- ½ red bell pepper, sliced

- ½ green bell pepper, sliced

- 2 kale leaves

- 1 C black beans, canned (rinsed)

- 3 tbsp. plain Greek-style yogurt

- 1 tsp. lemon juice

- 1 tsp. water

Instructions:

1. Preheat the oven to 425°F and place a big, rimmed baking sheet in the oven.

2. Combine the chili powder, cumin, salt, garlic powder, paprika, and freshly ground pepper in a large mixing bowl. 1 teaspoon of the spice combination should be transferred to a medium-sized mixing dish and put aside.

3. In a large mixing bowl, whisk oil into the remaining spice mixture. Toss in the chicken, onion, red and green bell peppers, and salt and pepper to taste.

4. Remove the pan from the oven and spray it with cooking spray to finish it. Using a spatula, evenly spread the chicken mixture over the pan. 15 minutes in the oven should be enough.

5. Place the kale and black beans in a large mixing dish with salt and olive oil. Toss to blend.

6. Turn off the oven and remove the pan. Combine the chicken and veggies in a large mixing bowl. Distribute the greens and beans on top in an equal layer. Continuing to roast for 5 to 7 minutes longer, or until the chicken is cooked through and soft veggies.

7. Combine the reserved spice combination with the yogurt, lime juice, and water – stirring constantly.

8. Distribute the chicken and vegetable mixture into four large mixing dishes. Finish by drizzling the yogurt dressing over the top and serving.

Nutritional Values:

Calories: 208kcal

Fat: 2.7g

Carbohydrates: 40g

Protein: 11g

Sodium: 288mg

13. Sweet Lentil Soup

Prep time: 10 mins

Cooking time: 30 mins

Serving: 2

Ingredients:

- 1 tsp. cumin powder

- 2 tsp. coriander seeds, crushed

- 1 onion, chopped

- 225g carrots, chopped

- 75gm red lentils

- 300ml orange-juice

- 2 tbsp. low-fat Greek-style yogurt

- Coriander and parsley for garnishing

- Paprika according to taste

- 600ml veggie or chicken stock

Instructions:

1. Crush coriander seeds in a crusher before roasting them in a big fry pan for 2 minutes or until light brown.

2. Bring carrots, lentils, onion, orange juice, vegetable stock, and spices to a boil in a large saucepan. Cover and cook for 30 minutes or until the lentils are tender.

3. Place it in a food processor in batches. Blend until a smooth paste is created.

4. Return it to the pan, re-heat over low heat, and stir lightly. Put everything into a separate serving plate and top with paprika and chopped coriander leaves.

Nutritional Values:

Calories: 356kcal

Fat: 2g

Carbohydrates: 40g

Protein: 14g

Sodium: 0.56g

14. Super Protein Bowl

Prep time: 15 mins

Cooking time: 40 mins

Serving: 2

Ingredients:

- 1 sweet potato, cut into standard size wedges

- ½ red onion, sliced thinly

- 1 tbsp. MCT oil

- ½ tsp. garlic powder

- ¼ tsp. pink salt, fine

- 8 oz. boneless chicken, cut into bite-sized chunks

- 2 tbsp. mustard sauce, fat-free

- 1 tbsp. maple syrup

- 1 tbsp. grape vinegar

- 4 C. green vegetables mixed, spinach, kale, iceberg

- ½ c. cooked quinoa of your choice

- 1 tbsp. Sunflower seeds or any seed of your choice.

Instructions:

1. Preheat the oven to 425°F. Combine sweet potato and onion with 1 tablespoon oil, garlic powder, and ⅛ teaspoon salt in a larger bowl.

2. Roast for 15 minutes, spreading evenly on a broad-rimmed baking sheet.

3. Combine chicken and 1 tablespoon mustard. Toss to coat. After 15 minutes, take the veggies from the oven and mix. Incorporate the chicken into the pan.

4. Return to the oven and continue roasting for approximately 10 minutes more, or until the veggies begin to brown and the chicken is cooked through. Allow to cool after removing from the oven.

5. In a large mixing bowl, whisk the maple syrup, vinegar, and the remaining 1 tablespoon oil, 1 tablespoon mustard, and ⅛ teaspoon salt.

6. When the chicken is cold enough to handle, shred it and add it to the bowl with the dressing. Combine the baby greens, quinoa, and roasted veggies in a large bowl.

7. Toss the salad with the dressing and top with sunflower seeds.

Nutritional Values:

Calories: 466kcal

Fat: 4g

Carbohydrates: 35.5g

Protein: 28g

Sodium: 715mg

Chapter 8: Other Tips and Tricks to Stay on Track

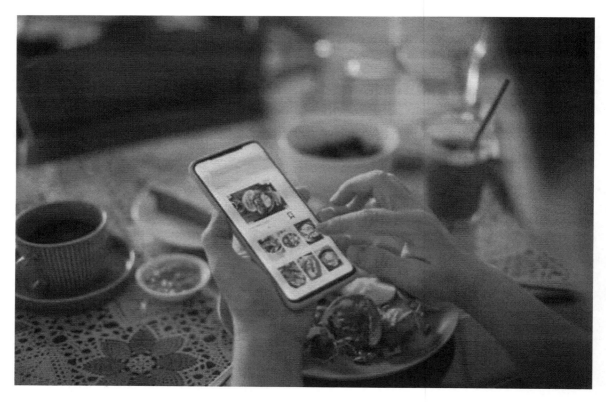

It does not matter how slowly you go, as long as you don't stop.

- As a substitute for cake, pie, or other sweets for dessert – try fresh fruit.

- Look after your physical appearance. When you've had your fill for the day, take a break from eating. Stop eating as soon as you feel full, satisfied, or sick from overindulging. You can have a little more if you're really hungry.

- Consume a high-fiber cereal daily.

- Consume a sufficient amount of fiber. Vegetables, fruits, and whole grains are excellent sources of vitamin A resulting in weight loss

- Consume food slowly. During meals, take a couple of one-minute pauses from chewing your food. Between nibbles, put your fork down on the table. Take little bites of your meal at a time.

- Dishes for serving should not be placed on the table. It will be more difficult to consume a second piece due to this.

- Don't forget to leave a little food on your plate. Remember that you have complete power over your diet; the food does not influence you.

- Drink a glass of water before you begin to eat your meal. Increase your fluid intake throughout meals.

- Drink lots of water or other calorie-free beverages (water, tea, coffee, diet soda). You may be thirsty rather than hungry.

- Eat at least three times every day to maintain your health.

- Instead of higher-fat/higher-calorie options, choose lean meats, low-fat or nonfat cheese, and skim (nonfat) or 1 percent fat milk.

- If you are still hungry or unsatisfied after eating a meal or snack, wait at least 10 minutes before eating again. Often, hunger will go away on its own.

- Keep all food items in the kitchen at all times. Only eat in a certain location, such as a dining room table.

- Make dinner a memorable occasion by serving it on beautiful plates, napkins, and glasses.

- Never eat in the vehicle, in your bedroom, or front of the television.

- Put the salad dressing on a plate to the side rather than mixing it into or pouring it over your salad. Take a fork and dip it into the dressing before spearing a mouthful of the salad.

- Rearrange your typical seating arrangement at the table.

- Reduce the number of alcoholic beverages (beer, wine, and liquor) that you consume.

- Reduce your intake of sugar. Drinking less fruit juice and ordinary soda may help you lose weight

- Remove your plate as soon as you finish eating. If you have leftovers that aren't going to be used, toss them away!

- Use smaller dishes, bowls, glasses, and serving spoons to provide a more intimate setting.

Chapter 9: 1200-Calories-A-Day 28-Day Meal Plan

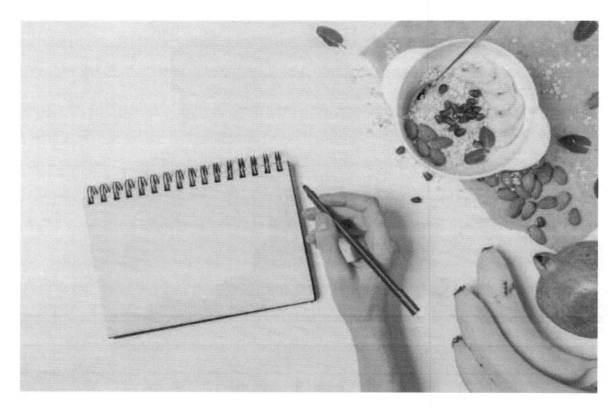

Planning your meals prevents poor decisions.

Day	Breakfast	Lunch	Dinner	Total Calories (kcal)
1	Breakfast Loaded Pepper	Tuna Kebabs	Barbequed Chicken	1220
2	Chia Pudding with Seasonal Fruits	Lentils Salad with Vegetables	Super Protein Bowl	1224
3	Protein Boost Bread	Honey Mustard Baked Chicken	Pork and Mushroom Gravy	1189

4	Berry-ola Yogurt Breakfast Bowl	Puy Lentils Burger	Super Protein Bowl	1166
5	Protein Pancakes	Sweet Potato Soup Curry	Roasted Asparagus with Potato and Chicken	1198
6	Scrambled Eggs	Kale Wraps with Turkey	Sweet Lentils Soup	1151
7	Choco Spinach Milk	Puy Lentils Burger	Barbequed Chicken	1128
8	Protein-Packed Breakfast Steak	Turkey Kofta	Tomato Pasta with Basil	1256
9	Slow Cook Breakfast Beans	Spinach with Apple Sauce Chicken	Black Lentils Soup	1204
10	Overnight Oats	Honey Mustard Baked Chicken	Red Lentils Soup	1192
11	Fruity Protein Bowl	Lemon Pepper Chicken Breasts	Super Protein Bowl	1126
12	Blueberry Turkey Kebabs	Sprouts Salad	Air Fryer Tofu Wrap	1410
13	Besan Pancake	Spinach with Apple Sauce Chicken	Pork and Mushroom Gravy	1145
14	Heavenly Tempeh Sandwich	Shrimp and Black Bean Salad	Turkey Patties	1218
15	Breakfast Loaded Pepper	White Fish with Stew	Pork and Mushroom Gravy	1139

16	Chia Pudding with Seasonal Fruit	Low Fat Spaghetti Squash	Barbequed Chicken	1187
17	Protein Boost Muffins	Sweet Potato Soup Curry	Roasted Asparagus with Chicken	1138
18	Berry-ola Yogurt Breakfast Bowl	Kale Wraps with Turkey	Super Protein Bowl	1161
19	Protein Pancakes	Tuna Kebabs	Ginger Chicken Korean style Bowl	1197
20	Protein-Packed Breakfast Steak	Cream of Chickpea Soup	Black Beans with Brown Rice	1193
21	Heavenly Tempeh Sandwich	White Fish with Stew	Shrimp and Corn Pasta	1193
22	Overnight Oats	Lemon Pepper Chicken Breast	Pork and Mushroom Gravy	1179
23	Choco Spinach Milk	Kale Wraps with Turkey	Sweet Lentils Soup	1131
24	Scrambled Eggs	Shrimp and Black Bean Salad	Super Protein Bowl	1200
25	Blueberry Turkey Kebabs	Spinach with Applesauce Chicken	Sweet Lentils Soup	1156
26	Fruity Protein Bowl	Honey Mustard Baked Chicken	Black Lentils Soup	1109

27	Besan Pancake	Honey Mustard Baked Chicken	Roasted Asparagus with Potato and Chicken	1144
28	Choco Spinach Milk	Sprouts Salad	Air Fryer Tofu Wrap	1240

Chapter 10: Body Recomposition and Metabolism

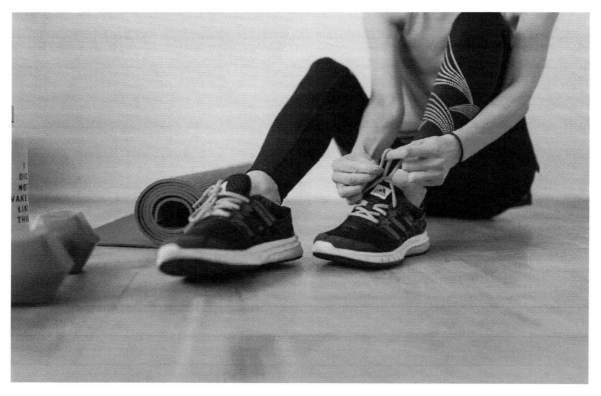

To change your body, you must first change your mind.

It is normal for a person to gain muscle while losing fat during the early stages of an exercise regimen. This is known as "body recomposition," and it becomes more difficult after the first phase, with most people having to alternate between bulking and reducing phases of their workouts. In reality, it is possible to maintain recomposition—that is, to continue gaining muscle while losing fat — for an extended period, at least until you are significantly slimmer and more muscular than the average person.

Getting rid of those extra pounds might cause your metabolism to slow down because you have less body weight to maintain. Our metabolism slows down as we shed excess pounds.

The process through which your body converts food into energy is known as metabolism. Think of it as a fire blazing in the furnace. It's always burning. Similarly, when you work out and eat correctly, you're adding fuel to it, causing it to burn to its fullest. We may do various things to slow our metabolism, including not eating enough, not eating regularly enough, and not moving enough. People who want to lose weight quickly and safely frequently use fad diets. Fad diets provide significant short-term benefits by significantly reducing calorie intake. These diets aren't meant to be long-term solutions as your metabolism will pick up speed at first, but then it will plummet dramatically.

To lose weight, you must limit your caloric intake. However, if you restrict your caloric intake too much, you may end up shooting yourself in the foot and not seeing the desired results in the long run.

So, to get started in the best way possible, you must first calculate your resting metabolic rate, which is the bare minimum of calories that we require if we do nothing but lie in bed all day. It contains enough calories to keep the heart pumping, the blood flowing, the lungs breathing, the body moving, and everything else going on.

Every time we eat, we get a slight increase in our metabolism, which is beneficial. Exercise provides a significant increase to our energy levels, particularly throughout that period. Strength training, in which you gain muscle mass, increases your resting metabolic rate because muscle consumes calories to maintain its shape.

Certain practices have been adopted from weight-loss success stories. Start each day with a healthy breakfast; eat a well-balanced, nutrient-dense, low-calorie, low-fat, protein-rich diet; exercise for at least an hour each day; and weigh yourself once a week to maintain a healthy metabolic rate and keep the weight off.

Chapter 11: The Next Step

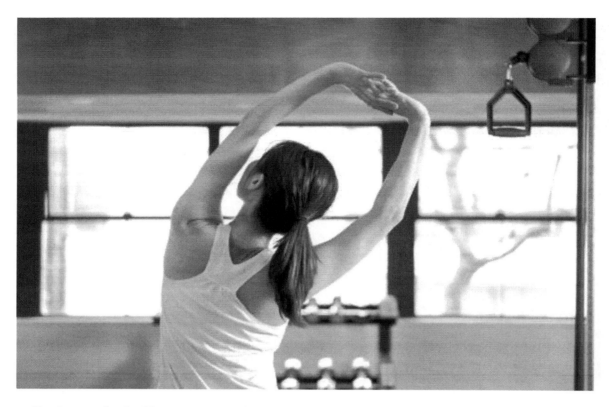

The most effective method of long-term weight reduction is to follow a sensible eating plan and exercise every day! You deserve to feel good in your body, and this note is just to wish you courage as you embark on your transformation and attainment of your goals.

The greatest diet is one that we can stick to for the rest of our lives, and it is just one component of a healthy lifestyle. According to the World Health Organization, aim for high-quality, nutritious whole meals that largely consist of plants (fruits and vegetables) while avoiding sugar, trans fats, and processed foods. It is advised that you engage in some form of physical activity, aiming for approximately two and a half hours of intense activity per week. Today, many people's healthy lifestyles include an improved stress management strategy and treatment for emotional disorders that may contribute to harmful eating behaviors.

Conclusion

Congratulations on gaining this valuable knowledge and learning about the best ingredients that your body will appreciate. You can now be your own boss and control your eating habits and diet. You won't be able to get enough of these recipes, and we made sure to please your taste buds as well.

Thank you for reading all the way through and making it to the end of this book. We hope you benefit your body and mind by eating healthy and that you never compromise on self-love, which is the key fuel to weight loss.